MEDICAL
TERMINOLOGY

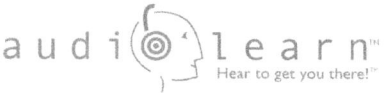

Table of Contents

Decoding Medical Terminology

Each area of expertise has its own "lingo" – lawyers use "legalese", pastors communicate in religious terms, bikers talk "Harley", and so on. To hike around in the health care field, you will have to know how to ask for directions, so to speak.

As health care professionals you will be expected to know the pronunciation and meaning of medical terms. Spelling counts, too, but you're on your own for that. These tapes will provide many of those terms more commonly used. Furthermore, we will give you a system that should help you figure out what almost any unfamiliar term means.

Medical terms are made up of root words, plus prefixes, suffixes, or both. Once you know the meaning of the parts, you can deduce the meaning of the entire term. Latin and Greek form the basis for most of the commonly used terms. If you have taken Spanish in school or Latin where it's still offered, you will recognize a good share of these prefixes, suffixes and root words.

For example, take the term **pericarditis** – it's made up of a prefix, **peri-** , meaning "surrounding"; the root word, **card-** , "the heart"; and a suffix, **-it is**, meaning "inflammation".

So we deduce that **pericarditis** means, "inflammation of the membrane surrounding the heart".

If you know the meaning of a word you are searching for, you can even construct it, sort of a do-it-yourself project, if you will.

Let's say you needed a term meaning, "an instrument used to inspect the cartilage inside a joint". You know the root for "an instrument used to inspect" is **scope**. From experience you will learn that "inside a joint" in this application does not mean the interior of a tavern, but is expressed by the prefix, **arthro-**.

Put them together and you have **arthroscope**.

The rest of this study package will present lists of commonly used root words, prefixes and suffixes, and finally, several hundred common terms. While these tapes are by no means a comprehensive listing, they will serve to familiarize you with the language you'll be using in your career.

Here is a list of **Root Words** and their meanings:

abdomin- , the abdomen, or the belly

acanth-, thorny, or spiny

acetabul-, the hip socket (acetabulum)

acou-, sound or hearing

acr-, extremities (for example, hands and feet), or height

actin-, radius, or ray (of light, possibly)

adenoid-, refers to the adenoids

aden-, resembling the adenoids or glandular tissue

adren-, refers to the adrenal gland

aer-, air, or gas

albumin-, the albumin

algesi-, pain

alveol-, alveolus

ambly-, dull, or dim

ambul-, walking

amni-, the amnion

amyl-, starch

andr-, male

angi-, vessel

antr-, antrum, a cavity or chamber

aort-, aorta

appendic-, the appendix

arachn-, spiders, or spiderlike

arche-, first, or beginning

arteri-, artery

arthr-, joint

articul-, joint, or hinge

ather-, yellowish, or fatty plaque (example: atherosclerosis)

atri-, atrium (of the heart)

aur-, ear, or hearing

aut-, self

axill-, armpit

azo-, urea or nitrogen

bacteri-, refers to bacteria

balan-, glans penis

bio-, life

bil-, the bile

blast-, a developing cell (as, blastomere)

blephar-, *(bleh-far)* eyelid

brach-, arm

bronch-, bronchus (part of the lung)

bucc-, cheek (of the face)

burs-, bursa (a cavity or sac)

calc-, calcium

carcin-, refers to cancer

cardi-, the heart

carp-, the carpals (wrist bones)

caud-, tail; toward the sacrum, where the tail would be on an animal

cec-, or **caec-**, *(seek-um)* cecum (or caecum), the first part of the large intestine

celi-, or **coeli-** (see-ly), the abdominal cavity

ceph-, relating to the brain

cerebell-, the cerebellum

cerebr-, cerebrum, or the brain itself

cerumin-, refers to cerumen, or earwax

cervic-, the dorsal part of the neck; or refers to a woman's cervix

chir-, hand

cholangi-, (ko-lan-jee) the bile duct

chol-, gall, or bile

choledoch-, (ko-le-doke) common bile duct

chondr-, cartilage

chori-, chorion

chrom-, color

clavic-, the clavicle (collarbone)

col-, the colon

colp-, refers to the vagina

coni-, dust

conjunctiv-, conjunctiva (the eye)

core-, (ko-ree) the pupil of the eye

corne-, the cornea

coron-, the heart

cortic-, cortex

cost-, rib

crani-, cranium (the skull)

cry-, cold

crypt-, hidden

cutane-, skin

cyan-, blue

cyst-, sac

cyt-, (site) cell

dactyl-, fingers or toes

dent-, tooth or teeth

derm-, skin

diaphor-, *(dye-a-for)* sweat

dips-, thirst

diverticul-, diverticulum

dors-, dorsal; in humans, the back (of the body)

duoden-, duodenum

ech-, sound

endocrin-, referring to the endocrine system

enter-, intestines

epididym-, *(ep-peh-**did**-im)* epididymis

epiglott-, the epiglottis

episi-, vulva

epitheli-, epithelium

erythr-, red

esophag-, esophagus

eti-, cause (of disease)

faci-, face

fasci-, fascia (a lining tissue)

febr-, fever

femor-, femur (upper leg bone)

fet-, fetus, or unborn child

fibr-, fibrous tissue; fibers

fibul-, fibula (lower leg bone)

fluor-, light

fung-, pertaining to fungus

gangl-, ganglion

gastr-, gastric; the stomach

ger-, elderly

gingiv-, the gums

gloss-, the tongue

gluc-, sugar

glyc-, carbohydrate or sugar (glucose)

gnath-, jaw

gon-, gonad, or sexual organ (male or female)

granul-, granulate (tissue around a wound during the healing process)

gyn-, woman

hem-, or **haem-**, *(heem)* the blood

hepat-, the liver

hern-, hernia

hist-, tissue

humer-, humerus (upper arm bone)

hybrid-, being a hybrid

hyster-, the uterus

ichthy-, fish

ile-, ileum (lower part of small intestine)

ili-, ilium (part of the pelvis)

immun-, immune

infarct-, refers to an infarct, or area of dead tissue from lack of oxygen

iri-, iris (of the eye)

ischi-, ischium (part of the pelvis)

lacr-, pertaining to tears

laryng-, refers to the larynx

lip-, fat

lymph-, referring to the lymph or lymphatic system

lysis-, lysis (can be used as root, prefix or suffix),

meaning destruction

macul-, macula (mack-you-lah)

mamm-, **mast-**, breast

mandibul-, the lower jawbone (mandible)

maxill-, the upper jawbone (maxilla)

membran-, membrane, covering

men-, **mens-**, referring to menstruation

ment-, the mind

morph-, form, or shape

muc-, mucus

myc-, fungus

myel-, pertains to myelin

myo-, muscle

nas-, **naso-**, the nose

nat-, birth

necr-, death (of cells or the body)

nephr-, kidney

neur-, nerve

noct-, **nyct-**, night

obstetr-, refers to obstetrics

ocul-, eye

olf-, olfactory (the sense of smell)

omphal-, the umbilicus, or navel

onc-, tumor

oo-, **ov-**, egg

oophor-, ovary

ophth-, eye

opt-, vision

orch-, testis

oste-, bone

ot-, ear

ox-, oxygen

pancr-, pancreas

papill-, nipple, or nipple-shaped

par-, **part-**, to bear, or give birth to

patell-, patella (the kneecap)

path-, disease

pector-, the chest

ped-, foot

ped-, **pedi-**, child

pelv-, pelvis, or pelvic bone

perine-, perineum

peritone-, peritoneum

petr-, stone

phag-, to eat or swallow

pharm-, pharmacy

pharyn-, pharynx or upper esophagus

phleb-, vein

phot-, light

phren-, the mind

plasm-, plasma

pleur-, pleura

pneum-, the lung; air

pod-, foot

proct-, rectum

prostat-, prostate gland

psych-, the mind

pulmon-, lung

py-, **pyelo-**, infection

radi-, radiation

rect-, rectum

ren-, kidney

respirat-, breathing

retin-, retina

rheumat-, refers to the musculoskeletal system, including the immune system

rhin-, nose

sacchar-, sugar

sacr-, sacrum, or "tailbone"

scler-, sclera (the"white" of the eye)

seb-, oil

sept-, septum

ser-, serum

soma-, body

somn-, sleep

son-, sound

splen-, the spleen

spondyl-, vertebra

tars-, tarsus (ankle bones)

tendin-, **tendon-**, refers to the tendons

test-, testicles or testis

thorac-, thorax or chest

thromb-, clot

thyr-, **thyroid-**, of the thyroid

tibi-, tibia (a lower leg bone)

trache-, trachea ("tray-kee-ah")

typh-, typhoid or typhus

urethr-, refers to the urethra

urin-, urine

uter-, uterus

uvul-, uvula (flap of tissue hanging down from the soft palate)

vaccin-, vaccine

vagin-, vagina

valv-, **valvul-**, valve

vas-, **vascul-**, vessel or duct

ven-, vein

ventricul-, relating to the ventricle

vertebr-, vertebra

vesic-, vesicle (or, small pouch)

vir-, virus

viscer-, the viscera (internal organs)

vulv-, vulva

Prefixes indicate position (*super-,* above), existing environmental considerations (*xeri-,* dry), location (*acro-,* top or summit), action (*ad-,* to or toward), amount (*milli-,* thousandth part of) and so on. Here is a listing of common **prefixes** and their meanings.

a-, an-, without, or absence of

ab-, from; away from

acro-, top; summit; furthest out; extremities, as arms or legs

ad-, to; toward

aer-, aero-, air

alb-, white

ana-, up; again; backward

ante-, before

anti-, against

api-, upon, or on top of

apo-, off

arachn-, spider

auto-, self

bi-, two

bio-, life

brachy-, short

centi-, hundredth part (as in, centimeter)

chemo-, chemical

co-, **con-**, with

contra-, against

cyto-, cell

de-, from; down; lack of

desmo-, fetter or band

dextro-, to the right

di-, two or double

dia-, through; throughout; completely

dis-, not; free from; to undo

dys-, inability; lack of

echo-, sound

eco-, environment

ect-, **ecto-**, outer; outside

electro-, using electricity

en-, **end-**, **endo-**, inside; within

entero-, the intestine; the gut

epi-, on, upon; at, by, near; over, on top of; toward; against; among

ergo-, work

eu-, goodly or well; also, normal

ex-, **exo-**, out of; outer; away from

extra-, outside of; beyond

ferro-, iron

fore-, in front of; ahead of

gastr-, the stomach

geno-, gene; genetic

gyn-, **gyne-**, **gyneco-**, **gyno-**, woman; womanlike; womanly

helic-, **helico-**, spiral

hemi-, half

hetero-, different

hex-, **hexo-**, six

histo-, tissue

homo-, same

hydro-, water; fluid

hyper-, above; excessive

hypn-, **hypno-**, sleep

hypo-, below; deficient; incomplete

iatr-, referring to a physician or to medicine

ichthy-, fish, fishlike

im-, into

in-, not; into

infra-, under; below

inter-, between

intra-, inside

ipsi-, the same

iso-, equal, or like

juxta-, near, nearby, close

karyo-, nucleus

kerato-, may refer to the cornea (e.g., keratitis) or to hard, horny tissue (e.g., keratosis)

keto-, ketone

kilo-, thousand (a kilogram is 1,000 grams)

lact-, milk; lactose

later-, side

lati-, width

leuk-, **leuko-**, literally, "white", refers to white blood cells

lip-, **lipo-**, fat

litho-, stone

longi-, length

lys-, **lyso-**, destroy, break apart

macro-, large, or long

mal-, bad or badly

mega-, great or huge; abnormally large

meso-, middle

meta-, after

micro-, small, or short

milli-, thousandth (there are 1,000 milligrams in a gram)

mono-, one or single

multi-, several; many

neo-, new, young, recent

nulli-, none

oligo-, just a few; scanty

omni-, all

omphal-, the umbilicus, or navel

onycho-, having to do with the nails

ortho-, straight, or erect (e.g., orthodontics, straightening the teeth)

osteo-, bones

oto-, ear

pachy-, elephant(like)

pan-, all

para-, beside, near; resembling; beyond; apart from; abnormal

patho-, suffering, or disease

per-, through

peri-, surrounding

phago-, (fay-go) devouring

phlebo-, vein

photo-, light

phys-, **physio-**, function

phyto-, plant

pneumo-, breathing, the lungs, pneumonia, or air

poly-, many

post-, after

pre-, before

pro-, before; in front of; preceding; on behalf of; in place of; the same as; initiating

pseudo-, false

quad-, quadr-, four; fourfold

quasi-, seemingly

re-, again

retro-, backward

schizo-, split; divided

sclero-, hard; or referring to the sclera of the eye

sub-, underneath

super-, above; before

supra-, upper

syn-, together

tachy-, speedy; too fast

tetra-, four

thrombi-, **thrombo-**, referring to a clot within a blood vessel or the heart

toc-, **toco-**, **tok-**, **toko-** referring to labor or childbirth

tox-, poisonous

trans-, over, across, beyond

tri-, three

ultra-, beyond, in excess

un-, not

uni-, one

xanth-, yellow

xen-, **xeno-**, foreign

xeri-, **xero-**, dry

zoo-, animal

zygo-, egg

Suffixes describe a procedure (*-ectomy,* removal), indicate action (*-phage,* consuming), relation (*-ous,* pertaining to), parts of the body (*-emia,* of the blood), and so on. They are elaborations on the root words, if you will. Here is a list of some common **suffixes** and their meanings.

-ac, -al, -ar, -ary, pertaining to

-agra, excessive pain

-algia, pain

-apheresis, removal

-ase, enzyme

-asthenia, weakness

-atresia, closure; occlusion; absence of a normal opening

-cele, -coele, (seel) hernia; protrusion

-centesis, surgical puncture to aspirate fluid

-cidal, killing

-clasia, -clasis, -clast, break

-clysis, irrigating or washing

-coccus, *(cock-us)* spherical, used in description of bacteria; plural is **cocci** *(cocks-eye)*

-crine, separate

-crit, to separate

-cyte, cell

-desis, surgical fixation, or fusion

-drome, running

-eal, **-ial**, pertaining to

-ectasis, dilatation; expansion; stretching out

-ectopia, displacement

-emesis, vomiting

-emia, **-aemia**, state of the blood

-er, one who

-esis, condition

-gen, substance or agent that causes (e.g., pathogen, something that causes disease)

-genesis, origin or cause

-genic, producing, causing

-gram, record, or x-ray film

-graph, record, or the device used to make such a record

-graphy, the process of recording

-ia, condition

-iatry, treatment of

-ic, pertaining to

-ician, one who treats or maintains (*physician*, one who treats the body)

-**ism**, state of

-**itis**, inflammation of

-**lepsy**, seizure

-**lysis**, breaking down; loosening; destruction (*bacteriolysis*, destruction of bacteria)

-**lyte**, subjected to decomposition (*electrolyte*, a solution that decomposes to ions and then conducts electricity)

-**lytic**, referring to lysis (*hemolytic*, the breakdown of red blood cells)

-**malacia**, softening

-**mania**, madness; obsessive desire

-**megaly**, enlargement

-**meter**, measuring device

-**metry**, measurement

-**morph**, form; shape

-**motor**, referring to motion

-**ness**, the state of

-**oid**, resembling

-**ologist**, one who studies

-ology, the study of

-oma, tumor; swelling

-opia, vision condition (myopia, nearsightedness)

-opsy, to view or examine (biopsy, to examine a sample of tissue)

-orrhagia, rapid flow of blood

-orrhaphy, suturing; repairing

-orrhea, flow; excessive discharge

-orrhexis, rupture

-osis, abnormal condition; increased (when used with blood cell root words)

-ostomy, creation of an artificial opening

-otomy, incision

-ous, pertaining to

-oxia, oxygen

-paresis, slight paralysis

-pathy, disease

-penia, abnormal reduction in number

-pepsia, digestion

-pexy, surgical fixation; suspension

-phagia, consuming; eating; swallowing

-philia, love

-phobia, abnormal fear

-**phonia**, sound; voice

-**phoria**, feeling

-**physis**, growth

-**plasia**, formation; development; growth

-**plasm**, a growth, substance or formation

-**plasty**, surgical repair

-**plegia**, paralysis

-**pnea**, breathing

-**poiesis**, formation

-**porosis**, full of passages (*osteoporosis*, passages in the bones)

-**prandial**, meal

-**praxia**, in front of; before

-**ptosis**, sagging; dropping; extrusion (prolapse)

-**ptysis**, spitting

-**scope**, instrument for visual examination

-**scopic**, -**scopy**, visual examination

-**sepsis**, infection

-**sis**, state of

-**spasm**, sudden involuntary muscle contraction

-**stalsis**, contraction

-**stasis**, control; stop

-**stenosis**, constriction; narrowing

-tome, a cutting instrument

-toxin, poison

-tripsy, surgical crushing

-trophy, nourishment

-ule, small

-uria, relating to urine

Some Common Medical Terms

Now that you have become acquainted with some of the root words, prefixes and suffixes, we'd like to introduce you to a grouping of medical terms that are used often. Using what you know, see if you can figure out the meanings before the narrator says them. Sorry, there's no prize at the end, except for your satisfaction in becoming familiar with some tools of your trade.

1. **abdomen** – lower part of the torso; the belly

2. **abduction** – taking away; the opposite of **adduction**, bringing toward

3. **abiotrophy** – loss of function, or degeneration, for unknown reasons

4. **abortifacient** – something that causes abortion

5. **abscission** – cutting away, as in surgery

6. **acanthamoeba** – *(a-**kanth**-a-mee-ba)* microorganism found in soil, dust, fresh water of all types, as well as HVAC units, humidifiers and dialysis units. Acanthamoeba enters the body through cuts, wounds, the nostrils or by swallowing and causes infection, especially to the central nervous system.

7. **acapnia** – lower than normal level of carbon dioxide in the blood

8. **achondroplasia** – *(a-kon-dro-**play**-zha)* genetic disorder of bone growth causing dwarfism

9. **acne vulgaris** – the kind of skin eruptions most commonly found in teens, caused by constriction of oil glands

10. **acrocyanosis** – blueness of the hands and feet, caused by constriction of the arterioles supplying blood to them

11. **acromegaly** – *(akro-**meg**-a-lee)* enlarged hands and feet, thickened skin and soft tissues; caused by too much human growth hormone

12. **acromioclavicular joint** – sliding joint located at the juncture of the point of the shoulder and the clavicle

13. **acupuncturist** – one who treats disease by controversial means of thin needles inserted into various parts of the body

14. **adenocarcinoma** – cancer that develops in the lining or inner surface of an organ

15. **adenoidectomy** – removal of the adenoids

16. **adenomyosis** – common condition in which the endometrium of the uterus grows into the myometrium

17. **adrenoleukodystrophy** – *(ad-ree-no-loo-ko-**dis**-tro-fee)* genetic disorder causing the breakdown of myelin sheath of nerve cells in the brain, with progressive dysfunction of the adrenal gland

18. **aerophobia** – fear of flying

19. **agammaglobulinemia** – absence of infection-fighting proteins in the blood; can be caused by HIV/AIDS

20. **agranulocytosis** – marked decrease of granulocytes (general infection-fighting cells in the blood)

21. **albuminuria** – greater than normal amount of albumin in urine

22. **alopecia** – baldness

23. **alveolus** (pl., **alveoli**) – *(al-vee-o-lus/lie)* tiny sac at the end of a bronchiole in the lung

24. **amenorrhea** – *(ay-men-o-ree-a)* cessation of menstruation

25. **amyloidosis** – disease resulting from abnormal deposits of amyloid protein in various parts of the body

26. **analgesic** – relieving pain

27. **anaphylaxis** – allergic reaction

28. **anesthesiology** – study and practice of the use of drugs or other agents that cause insensibility to pain

29. **aneurysm** – bulge in the wall of a blood vessel or the heart

30. angina – chest pain arising from inadequate supply of oxygen to the heart because of an embolus

31. **angioedema** – red, itchy, irritated areas in the skin; similar to hives but in deeper layers

32. **anhydrosis** – *(an-high-**dro**-sis)* too little sweating (do not confuse with **anhidrosis**, *(an-hid-**ro**-sis)* no sweating)

33. **anomaly** – deviation from the norm

34. **anophthalmia** – *(an-off-**thal**-mee-a)* congenital absence of the eye

35. **anorexia** – decreased appetite due to aversion to food

36. **anoxia** – lack of oxygen

37. **antenatal** – before birth

38. **anteroposterior** – from front to back, as in x-ray technique

39. **antibacterial** – something that inhibits or destroys bacteria

40. **anticoagulant** – a substance that prevents blood from clotting

41. **aphagia** – inability to eat

42. **aphasia** – literally, "no speech"; may apply either to the inability to express or to understand

43. **aphrasia** – inability to speak phrases or to understand them

44. **apiphobia** – fear of bees

45. **apoptosis** – programmed cell death, occurs normally to systematically replace old cells

46. **apraxia** – inability to move, despite normal muscle function; caused by a dysfunction in the cortex of the brain

47. **arachnoiditis** – inflammation of the middle layer of membranes covering the brain and spinal cord

48. **arbovirus** – ARthropod BOrne virus; one transmitted by mosquitos, ticks, etc. (note: this virus has nothing to do with trees, so its name is NOT **arbor**virus)

49. **arrhythmia** (note: this is spelled with 2 'r's) – abnormal heartbeat

50. **arteriogram** – x-ray of the blood vessels

51. **arteriosclerosis** – hardening and thickening of the artery walls

52. **arthritis** – inflammation of a joint

53. **arthrocentesis** – using a sterile needle and syringe to draw fluid from a joint

54. **arthroscopy** – inserting a small tube into a joint to view, diagnose and repair tissues (do not confuse with orthoscopy – correction of vision)

55. **aseptic** – absence of microorganisms; sterile

56. **asphyxia** – impaired breathing

57. **aspiration** – removal of fluid or cells through a needle; also, accidental ingestion of fluid or particles into the lungs

58. **astigmatism** – blurring or part of an image because of irregular curvature of the eye

59. **atherosclerosis** – progressive deposit of plaque on the inside walls of arteries, resulting in coronary artery disease or stroke

60. **atrioventricular** – referring to both the upper and lower chambers of the heart

61. **auscultation** – *(oss-kull-tay-shun)* listening via stethoscope to the internal organs

62. **axillary** – *(ax-il-air-ee)* pertaining to the armpit (do not confuse with **auxiliary** – *(awk-zil-yair-ee)* in addition to)

63. **azoospermia** – *(ay-zoe-oh-sper-mee-ah)* no sperm cells at all

64. **azotemia** – higher than normal level of urea or nitrogen compounds in the blood, usually caused by the inability of the kidney to excrete them

65. **Babinski reflex** – (normally found in infants) a blunt object or the thumb drawn from heel to toes on the sole of the foot produces an extension of the great toe and fanning of the others

66. **bacillus** – *(ba-sill-us)* any of a family of rod-shaped bacteria

67. **bacteremia** – presence of bacteria in the blood

68. **bacteriophage** – a virus living inside a bacterium (be careful! *Phage* does not always mean "to eat")

69. **balanitis** – inflammation of the head of the penis

70. **balanoposthitis** – in uncircumcised males, inflammation of both the head of the penis and the foreskin

71. **barosinusitis** – discomfort of the sinuses due to a change in altitude or barometric pressure (commonly experienced in airplanes on takeoff or landing)

72. **bathophobia** – fear of depths

73. **bicarbonate** – short for "bicarbonate of soda" (baking soda), used to neutralize indigestion

74. **bicuspid** – literally, "two flapped"

75. **biliary atresia** – *(billy-airy a-tree-zha)* congenital absence or closure of bile ducts

76. **bilirubin** – *(bill-a-roo-bin)* yellow-orange compound produced normally by the breakdown of hemoglobin from red blood cells

77. **biological** – of life

78. **blepharospasm** – *(bleff-a-ro-spazm)* involuntary, forcible closure of the eyelids

79. **brachial plexus** – a bundle of nerves going from the back of the neck and extending through the axilla

80. **brachycephaly** – *(bracky-seff-a-lee)* a short head from front to back, resulting in "moon face"; generally seen in Down syndrome

81. **bradycardia** – *(braddy-car-dee-ah)* slow heart rate, usually less than 60 beats per minute

82. **bronchopulmonary** – relating to the air passages of both the bronchi and the lung itself

83. **brucellosis** – "undulant fever"; transmitted by Brucella bacteria through infected dairy products, ungulates (split-hoofed animals) or their carcasses

84. **bruxism** – grinding or gnashing of teeth

85. **bulimia** – insatiable appetite, often accompanied by self-induced vomiting

86. **bursitis** – inflammation of the bursa, a fluid-filled sac that provides lubrication between tissues

87. **cadaver** – a deceased body used for the study of anatomy, the discovery of disease sites, detection of cause of death, or to provide tissue to repair a living human being

88. **caecum (cecum)** – *(seek-um)* first part of the large intestine

89. **calcaneus** – the heel bone

90. **calcinosis** – abnormal deposit of calcium salts in body tissues

91. **calcitonin** – hormone produced by the thyroid that lowers blood levels of calcium and phosphate, and promotes formation of bone

92. **campylobacteriosis** - the leading cause of bacterial food poisoning, most often spread by contact with raw or undercooked poultry

93. **Candida albicans** - yeast like fungal organism found in small amounts in the normal human

intestinal tract, usually kept in check by the rest of the microorganism community there

94. **candidiasis** - overgrowth of the C. albicans yeast in the gastrointestinal tract (bot not limited to that location)

95. **capitation** – a fixed amount that will be paid to a US health service provider per patient ("per capita")

96. **carbohydrate** – literally, "carbon and water"; mainly sugars and starches, these compounds are made up of carbon, hydrogen and oxygen in the proportion of one atom of carbon to one molecule of water $[C_n(H_2O)_n]$

97. **carcinoembryonic antigen** – (CEA) used mainly as a tumor marker for an indication of malignity; CEA is produced by some cancers ("carcino-") and by the developing fetus ("-embryonic")

98. **carcinogenic** – causing cancer

99. **carcinoma** - a cancer that begins in the tissues which line or cover an organ

100. **cardiomyopathy** - disease of the heart muscle

101. **cardiopulmonary** – referring to both the heart and lungs

102. **cardiovascular** – the blood vessels of the heart

103. **carotenemia** – harmless, temporary yellowing of the skin due to excess beta carotene in the diet

104. **catheterization** – use of a thin, flexible tube; in the circulatory system, insertion of a tiny tube (a

catheter) into a vein to deliver fluids or medication; in the urinary system, insertion of a tube into the bladder to drain urine

105. **cauterization** - using heat to destroy abnormal cells (also, "diathermy" or "electrodiathermy")

106. **celiac sprue** – *(see-lee-ack **sproo**)* result of an immune reaction to gluten, a protein found in wheat and many of the foods we eat; treatment is avoidance of foods containing gluten

107. **centimeter** – (abbrev., **cm**) one-hundredth of a meter; there are 2.54 cm in one inch

108. **centromere** - specialized region of the chromosome to which spindle fibers attach during cell division

109. **cephalic** – of the head

110. **cephalothoracic lipodystrophy** – *(seff-a-low-tho-**rass**-ick lippo-**dis**-tro-fee)* painless, symmetrical deposits of fat beneath the skin of the neck, upper trunk, arms and legs.

111. **cerebrospinal** – *(serree-bro-**spy**-nal)* of the head and spine

112. **cerebrovascular ferrocalcinosis** – *(serree-bro-**vass**-kyu-lar fair-o-kal-sin-**o**-sis)* Fahr's disease, a genetic neurological disorder that manifests abnormal deposits of calcium in certain parts of the brain

113. **cervical vertebra** – one of the vertebrae in the neck

114. **cheiroarthropathy** – *(kerro-arth-**rop**-ath-ee)* thickening of the skin causing contracture of the fingers, seen in diabetic patients

115. **chemokinesis** – *(kee-mo-kin-ee-sis)* "chemical movement", using a chemical to cause a cell to make changes in its movement by slowing down, speeding up or changing direction

116. **cholecystitis** – *(kola-sis-tie-tiss)* inflammation of the gallbladder, as a complication of gallstones

117. **cholestasis** – *(kola-stay-sis)* stagnant flow of bile from the liver

118. **cholesterol** – the most common type of steroid in the body, critical in development of bile acids, vitamin D, estrogens, androgens and certain hormones; cholesterol is also important in maintaining normal function of cell membranes

119. **chondroplasia** – formation of cartilage

120. **chondrosarcoma** – a cancer that forms in cartilage

121. **chorea** – "dancing", a rapid series of body movements that appear planned but are involuntary

122. **chorion** – the outer membrane that envelops the fetus; the placenta develops from the chorion

123. **choroid** – the thin middle layer of the eye between the sclera and the retina; the iris (colored part of the eye) is part of the choroid layer

124. **chromatography** – a laboratory technique used to separate and identify mixtures of substances

125. **cirrhosis** – *(sear-row-sis)* irreversible scarring of the liver; cirrhosis can occur because of alcohol, viral hepatitis B or C, and presently transplant appears to be the only option in advanced cases

126. **claudication** – limping

127. **clinodactyly** – curving of the little finger toward the ring finger

128. **Clostridium** – a family of anaerobic bacteria, which thrive in conditions without air; some of them wreak major havoc in human intestines, notably C. difficile and C. perfringens

129. **coccygeal vertebrae** – *(cock-sidge-ee-al)* the vertebrae that make up the coccyx, *(cock-six)* or "tail bone"

130. **coitus interruptus** – also called "withdrawal"; a method of birth control in which the man withdraws before ejaculation, its effectiveness depends on proper timing (in cases where this is the only form of contraception, there is no penalty for early withdrawal)

131. **colitis** – inflammation of the colon

132. **coloboma** - birth defect in which part of the eye does not form due tobecause of failure of the introcular fissure to properly close during embryonic development

133. **colorectal** – in the area of the colon and the rectum

134. **colostomy** – an alternative exit from the colon made by forming a hole therein and routing the contents through a tube in the abdominal wall, most often into a bag

135. **comedo** – "blackhead", formed by a blockage of a sebaceous gland

136. **condyloma subcutaneum** – *(kon-dill-**oh**-ma sub-kew-**tay**-nee-um)* wartlike growths around the anus and genitals caused by a virus.

137. **congenital** – from birth

138. **conjuncitivis** – inflammation of the conjunctiva of the eye

139. **consanguinity** – common ancestry

140. **contraceptive** – preventer of conception

141. **contraindication** – warning sign against a particular course of action or treatment

142. **contralateral** – on the other side

143. **contusion** – bruise

144. **coprolalia** – excessive, uncontrollable use of obscene language, particularly terms referring to bowel functions; often occurs as a part of Tourette syndrome

145. **coronary angiography** – x-ray of the coronary arteries done from inside by means of a fluoroscope

146. **corpus callosum** - the area of the brain which connects the two cerebral hemispheres

147. **corticosteroid** - steroid hormones made by the cortex (outer layer) of the adrenal gland

148. **cortisone** – a naturally occurring hormone that is also widely synthesized for treatment of inflammation sites and adrenocortical deficiency

149. **coryza** – a head cold

150. **costochondritis** – inflammation of the rib cartilage

151. **coxa valga** – inward curvature of the hip

152. **cranial arteritis** – inflammation of the walls of the blood vessels in the head; also known as "temporal arteritis"

153. **craniometaphyseal dysplasia** - genetic skeletal condition that involves abnormal bone formation and overmineralization of the skull and the long bones

154. **craniotomy** – surgically opening the skull

155. **creatine** - a compound the body makes and then uses to store energy; synthetic creatine is sold as a dietary supplement used by athletes as a "legal steroid" to increase muscle bulk, but long-term safety of this usage is in question

156. **creatinine** - chemical waste molecule, produced from creatine, that is generated from muscle metabolism; valuable as an indicator of kidney function

157. **Crohn enterocolitis** – Crohn's disease involving only the small intestine

158. **cruciate ligament, anterior/posterior** – cartilage arrangement that holds the patella in place and allows the knee to flex

159. **cryoglobulin** - abnormal blood protein precipitates from the blood serum when it is chilled ("cryo-") and redissolves upon warming

160. **cryosurgery** – surgery performed using extremely low temperatures

161. **cryptorchidism** – a condition in which neither of the testes descend into the scrotum, but remain inside the body cavity; cryptorchid males are at greater risk for testicular cancer

162. **culdocentesis** - puncture of the cul-de-sac and aspiration of fluid from it (the cul-de-sac, the rectouterine pouch (the pouch of Douglas), is an extension of the peritoneal cavity between the rectum and back wall of the uterus)

163. **cutaneous** – of the skin

164. **cystitis** – inflammation of the bladder

165. **cystoscopy** – inspection of the interior of the bladder through a small tube inserted therein

166. **dactyledema** – swelling of the fingers and/or toes

167. **decongestant** – an agent used to relieve stuffiness of the nose and/or sinuses by shrinking the swollen membranes

168. **defibrillation** - use of a tightly controlled electric shock to restart or normalize heart rhythms; may be administered either by means of a device on the outside of the chest wall or directly to the exposed heart muscle

169. **demyelination** – removal of the myelin sheath from nerves

170. **dermabrasion** – surgically rubbing off the top layer of skin with sandpaper or other methods, to remove

small scars (*e.g.,* from acne), moles, tattoos or fine wrinkles

171. **dermatitis** – inflammation of the skin

172. **dermatologist** – one who studies and treats disorders of the skin

173. **desmoplasia** – the growth of fibrous or connective tissue

174. **desquamation** – normal shedding of the outer layers of skin

175. **dextrocardia** – the right side of the heart

176. **diabetes mellitus** – (or, simply, **diabetes**) a disorder caused by absence or insufficient production of insulin, yielding elevated levels of sugar in the blood; diabetes affects all systems in the body and should therefore be taken seriously; besides treatment with insulin and diet, exercise and weight loss are recommended as beneficial to diabetes patients

177. **dialysis** – removing excess waste materials from the blood due to the inability of the kidneys to excrete such waste

178. **diaphragm** – the muscle used for breathing, located in the torso just below the lungs; or, any thin, flat membrane

179. **diarrhea** – loose, sometimes explosively emitted, stool; can be a symptom of disease or simply too many peaches

180. **diastole** – *(dye-ass-to-lee)* the time the heart relaxes

181. **diastolic** – *(dye-ah-**stall**-ick)* referring to the time during the heartbeat cycle when the heart relaxes

182. **diathermy** – use of heat to destroy abnormal cells (also called cauterization)

183. **diethylstilbestrol** – DES; the first synthetic form of estrogen, it was widely prescribed in the 1950s and 60s to prevent miscarriages and premature births, but was later found to cause reproductive system abnormalities in the "DES babies", including a greater risk of cervical and uterine cancer

184. **dilatation** – enlargement or expansion, as the opening of the pupil of the eye via drops

185. **dilation** – same as dilatation

186. **dioxin** - any of a number of poisonous petrochemicals, produced when herbicides are made or when plastics are burned

187. **diphtheria** – *(diff-**theer**-eeyah)* caused by bacterial infection (Corynebacterium diphtheriae), this acute disease begins with a sore throat and mild fever, then rapidly proceeds to include the entire upper respiratory tract; very dangerous in children, it is one of the "Big 3" included in the usual DPT vaccination (diphtheria-pertussis-tetanus)

188. **dipsophobia** – abnormal fear of drinking alcohol

189. **distichiasis** – double rows of eyelashes

190. **diuretic** – an agent that removes excess water from the body through the kidneys

191. **diurnal** – active during the day (as opposed to nocturnal, active during the night)

192. **diverticulitis** – infection of the diverticula (pockets) of the large intestine

193. **diverticulosis** – the condition of having developed diverticula in the colon, may lead to diverticulitis if constipation is a problem

194. **dorsal** – referring to the back

195. **ductus arteriosus** – an arterial shunt in the fetus, where blood pumped from the heart through the pulmonary artery toward the lungs is diverted into the aorta; normally the ductus arteriosus closes by itself, but in premature births it may still be open and add to complications from respiratory stress syndrome

196. **duodenum** – the first part of the small intestine, where peptic ulcers are found most often

197. **dysentery** – inflammation of the intestine, with accompanying pain, diarrhea, bloody stools and so on; caused by an amoeba

198. **dyskinesia** – the presence of involuntary movements, such as in chorea

199. **dyslexic** – switching numbers or letters, either in reading or writing (example: The dyslexic atheist spent years denying the existence of Dog.)

200. **dyspeptic** – pertaining to dyspepsia, a general feeling of stomach upset or bloating

201. **dyspraxia** – impaired or painful function of any organ in the body

202. **dystocia** – abnormal or difficult labor or delivery

203. **dystonia** - involuntary movements and/or prolonged muscle contraction, resulting in twisting body motions, tremor, or abnormal posture; may be caused by something as simple as writer's cramp

204. **dystrophy** – weakening or abnormal development of muscle

205. **dysuria** – pain or difficulty when urinating

206. **echocardiography** - a diagnostic test using ultrasound waves to make images of the heart chambers, valves and surrounding structures for purposes of measuring heart output

207. **eclampsia** - convulsions occurring only with pregnancy-associated high blood pressure

208. **ectopic** – in the wrong place

209. **eczema** – skin irritation including (but not limited to) itching, burning, redness, bumps, blisters, roughening and scaling

210. **edema** – swelling because of fluid accumulation in the tissues

211. **efferent** – carrying away; an *efferent* nerve carries impulses away from the brain to other parts of the body; arteries are *efferent* blood vessels (opposite: **afferent**, carrying toward)

212. **effusion** – too much fluid, or an outpouring of the same

213. **eisoptrophobia** – fear of mirrors

214. **electrocardiogram** – using electric current to show a continuous graph of the heart rhythm; commonly called an EKG

215. **electrolysis** – permament removal of body hair with an electronic tool

216. **electrophoresis** - procedure used in laboratories for separating molecules according their size and electrical charge, notably large molecules such as DNA fragments or proteins, from a mixture of molecules

217. **embolism** – the condition of having an embolus, or blood clot

218. **emesis** – vomiting

219. **emphysema** – *(em-fizz-ee-mah)* most commonly, a lung condition associated with smoking, caused by abnormal accumulation of air in the lung's many tiny air sacs (alveoli), which causes them to break and no longer be able to function; emphysema victims literally suffocate

220. **empyema** - *(em-pye-em-ah)* pus in the pleural space (between the outer surface of the lung and the chest wall), often a complication of bacterial pneumonia or type B influenza

221. **encephalitis** – inflammation of the brain, can occur as a complication of measles

222. **encephalomyelitis** – inflammation of both the brain and spinal cord, also called *myeloencephalitis*

223. **endocardium** – interior lining of the heart, consisting of a layer of endothelial cells outside a layer of connective tissue

224. **endocrine** – relating to hormones, their production and the diseases that affect the endocrine system

225. **endogenous** – inside; for instance, cholesterol is endogenous (made inside the body) and vitamin C is not (do not confuse with *indigenous*, naturally occurring in the surroundings)

226. **endometrial** – referring to the inner lining of the uterus (endometrium); this is the layer that accumulates and then is shed during each menstrual cycle

227. **endometriosis** – a condition of women during the childbearing years in which cells that normally are found inside the uterus migrate outside and implant themselves in various sites, usually throughout the abdominal cavity; there may be pain associated, or no apparent symptoms; endometriosis may cause infertility if the growth occurs in the fallopian tubes, but there does not appear to be an increased risk of cancer

228. **endorphin** – a painkiller manufactured by the body itself, in the brain, spinal cord, or elsewhere

229. **endoscopy** – examination of the interior of the body via a lighted tube, usually inserted through a natural opening (mouth or anus)

230. **endothelium** – inner lining of flat cells in the blood vessels, lymphatic vessels, and heart

231. **endotracheal** – inside the trachea

232. **enteritis** – inflammation of the small intestine

233. **enterobiasis** – pinworm infection, caused by Enterobius vermicularis; pinworms live and reproduce in the skin around the anus

234. **enterocolitis** – inflammation of both the small and large intestine

235. **enteropathy** – disease of the small intestine

236. **enterospasm** – painful, intense contraction of the intestine

237. **enterovirus** - a virus that enters the body through the gastrointestinal tract, often moving on to attack the nervous system; the polioviruses, rhinoviruses, and echoviruses are all enteroviruses

238. **enuresis** – involuntary urination, including but not limited to bed-wetting

239. **eosinophil** – a kind of white blood cell having coarse granules within its cytoplasm, which often increases in numbers in the presence of an allergic reaction

240. **epicardium** – the outer layer of heart tissue

241. **epidemiology** – the study and treatment of outbreaks of disease

242. **epidermoid carcinoma** – also called squamous cell carcinoma, this is a type of lung cancer where the cells are flat and resemble fish scales

243. **epididymus** - a coiled segment of the spermatic ducts that serves to store, mature and transport sperm between the testis and the vas deferens

244. **epigastric** – that part of the abdomen above the umbilicus

245. **epiglottis** – the flap covering the trachea during swallowing to prevent intrusion into the lungs

246. **epilation** – removal of body hair by a variety of methods, including electrolysis, tweezers or wax; sometimes performed by a dermatologist, but usually by a cosmetician (also called *depilation*)

247. **epilepsy** - a pattern of repeated seizures, may be caused by blows to the head, fever, or inherited disorder

248. **epinephrine** – (synonym: adrenaline) a substance produced inside the adrenal gland as part of the fight-or-flight reaction, which quickens heartbeat, strengthens the force of the heart's contraction and opens up the bronchioles in the lungs, among other things; epinephrine is widely used as an antidote to bee stings among those allergic to bee venom

249. **episiotomy** – during childbirth, an intentional cut of the mother's skin between the vulva and anus, to prevent a possibly more serious tear that could involve the rectum

250. **epithelium** - the outer layer of cells covering all surfaces of the body including the skin, plus the

mucous membranes that are continuations of the skin (*e.g.,* the lining of the mouth and nose)

251. **ergonomics** – the study of the surroundings of work and how they affect the body (posture, repetitive actions, and so on)

252. **erythema** – redness of the skin caused by inflammation, as in sunburn or lupus

253. **erythrocyte** – a red blood cell

254. **erythromycin** – a common antibiotic used to treat bacterial infections such as pneumonia

255. **Escherichia coli** – a bacillus that occurs naturally in the colon; however, if ingested from outside sources a particular strain of E. coli can wreak havoc with the intestine via "food poisoning"

256. **esophagus** – the tube between the mouth and the stomach

257. **esophagogastroduodenoscopy** – *(ee-soff-ah-go-gas-tro-doo-odd-en-os-cop-ee)* easy for YOU to say! - a procedure that allows examination of the esophagus, stomach and duodenum (first part of the small intestine), using a thin flexible tube (but please, put me to sleep first!)

258. **estrogen** – a female hormone produced by the ovaries, lack of which can cause osteoporosis

259. **eugenics** - literally, "normal genes", eugenics aims to improve the genetic constitution of the human species by selective breeding; this is also known as meddling

260. **euphoria** – a feeling of superlative well-being

261. **euthanasia** – "assisted death"

262. **exophthalmos** – protruding eyes, typical of hyperthyroidism

263. **extracorporeal shock wave lithotripsy** – a non-invasive procedure designed as an alternative to surgery to break up gallstones or kidney stones using shock waves

264. **extubation** – removal of a tube, often from the airway; opposite of **intubation**

265. **exudative angina** – (also called *angina trachealis*, more commonly known as **croup**) infection of the larynx, trachea, and bronchial tubes, occurring mainly in children and caused by viruses and, sometimes, bacteria; characterized by a barking cough and a harsh gasp during inhaling

266. **fallopian tube** – the tube leading from the ovary to the uterus, through which a woman's egg travels during her monthly cycle

267. **fascia** – lining tissue under the skin that covers a variety of surfaces and also encases muscles

268. **fasciculation** - involuntary contractions or twitchings of groups of muscle fibers; may occur for no apparent reason or as a result of illness

269. **femoral** – referring to the femur, or thigh bone

270. **fenestration** – literally, "making a window", constructing a new opening

271. **fetoscopy** – procedure for examination of a baby while yet inside the womb

272. **fibrillation** – uncoordinated twitching of the heart muscle, not the same as flutter, which is organized and normal

273. **fibrinogen** – the protein from which fibrin is formed during normal blood clotting

274. **fibroid** – a benign tumor of the uterus, the most common indication for hysterectomy

275. **fibromyalgia** – (also known as *fibrositis*) chronic pain, stiffness and tenderness of muscles, tendons and joints without obvious inflammation; no body damage or deformity is caused, but persistent fatigue and insomnia accompany this condition

276. **fibula** – the outside bone of the lower leg (the inside bone is the *tibia*)

277. **filovirus** – a family of viruses, such as Ebola virus, which cause hemorrhagic fever

278. **fissure** – a crack

279. **fistula** – an abnormal passageway

280. **flatus/flatulence** – the production and emission of gas in the stomach or intestine; also known as belching or farting

281. **flavivirus** – a family of viruses transmitted by mosquitoes and ticks that cause hemorrhagic fever; yellow fever is caused by a flavivirus

282. **fluorescein angiography** – a test to examine blood vessels in the retina, choroid layer and iris of the eye, by injecting a special dye into a vein in the arm; pictures are then taken as the dye passes through the blood vessels in the eye, to detect various diseases, especially macular degeneration

283. **fluorouracil** – an anticancer drug

284. **fontanel (fontanelle)** – the "soft spot" in a baby's skull where the cranial plates have not yet grown together

285. **foramen** (pl., **foramina**) – a naturally occurring opening, usually in bone

286. **forensic** - dealing with the application of scientific knowledge to legal problems, especially where a crime has been committed or is suspected

287. **formaldehyde** – a colorless, poisonous gas which, when put into aqueous solution, is used for disinfecting and preservation of tissues

288. **fornix** (pl., **fornices**) – a vaultlike or arched structure, usually connecting two larger ones

289. **furuncle** – otherwise known as a boil

290. **fusospirillosis** – *trenchmouth*; this disease has been around a long time, but its causes are not easy to pin down, therefore it is known as a variety of horrible-sounding forms of gingivitis (go get your teeth cleaned today!)

291. **galactosemia** – a buildup of galactose (a sugar) in the blood, resulting from an inability to metabolise lactose (milk sugar); exposure to any kind of milk

(human or otherwise) or milk products will cause liver damage, mental retardation, cataract formation, and kidney failure

292. **gametogenesis** – production of sexual reproductive cells

293. **gastrectomy** – removal of part or all of the stomach

294. **gastritis** – inflammation of the stomach

295. **gastroesophageal reflux** – backup of stomach contents into the esophagus, often causing heartburn (also called acid reflux)

296. **gastroschisis** - a birth defect in which part of the intestines protrude through a separation of the abdominal wall to one side of the umbilicus, and are not covered by the peritoneum

297. **genitourinary** – referring to the genitals and the urinary tract

298. **gestation** – the time needed for a baby to develop, from conception to birth

299. **gingivitis** – inflammation of the gums

300. **ginkgo biloba** – a large ornamental tree of Chinese origin, having fan-shaped leaves; ginkgo is used in herbal supplements to increase concentration and sharpen mental acuity, presumably by causing increased circulation in the brain

301. **glans penis** – the rounded head of the penis

302. **glaucoma** – increased pressure within the eye; cause is unknown and there is no cure, but early detection

is valuable for treatment to arrest the progress of the condition, which if left to itself will cause blindness

303. **glioblastoma multiforme** – a very malignant type of brain tumor arising from glial cells (the connective tissue of the central nervous system); early symptoms include sleepiness, headache, and vomiting

304. **globus** – literally, a globe or sphere; globus may refer to a number of things, among them: *globus hystericus* (or simply globus), the feeling of having a lump in one's throat; *globus major* and *globus minor*, structures in the epidydimus; and *globus pallidus*, a rounded whitish area in the brain

305. **glossolalia** – nonsense sounds that mimic understandable speech, often experienced during sleep or while "speaking in tongues"

306. **glottis** – a flap in the larynx that covers the vocal cords

307. **glucosamine** - a molecule which results from the addition of an amino group to glucose; naturally occurring in the blood and in cartilage, glucosamine as a nutritional supplement may improve symptoms of pain and stiffness in some osteoarthritis patients

308. **gluteus maximus** – the large muscle in the buttocks

309. **glycoprotein** – any of a group of key molecules made of a carbohydrate plus a protein; in an immune response, for example, nearly all of the molecules most important are glycoproteins

310. **gonadotropin** - hormones secreted by the pituitary gland which affect the function of the male or female reproductive organs

311. **gonorrhea** - an infectious STD (sexually transmitted disease) caused by bacteria which can also be transmitted to the newborn during birth; half of all women infected with gonorrhea experience no symptoms, which contributes to its proliferation

312. **granulocyte** – a type of white blood cell filled with tiny granules which on closer inspection prove to be sacs filled with enzymes to aid in disposing of any foreign entities taken in by the cell

313. **granulomatous colitis** – Crohn's disease of the colon

314. **gynecoid** – womanlike

315. **gynecologist** – one who treats the reproductive systems of women

316. **Helicobacter pylori** – the most common cause of stomach ulcers in the world, H. pylori is a bacteriun causing stomach inflammation (gastritis) which leads to ulcers

317. **hemangioma** – when visible through the skin, commonly known as a "birthmark"; a birth irregularity where an area of tissue becomes rich in small blood vessels

318. **hematocrit** - the proportion of the blood that consists of red blood cells, packed by centrifugation, expressed as a percentage of volume

319. **hematologist** – one who treats conditions of the blood

320. **hematopoiesis** – development of blood cells

321. **hemiplegia** – literally, "half-paralyzed"; afflicted by the loss of function in any two of one's arms and/or legs

322. **hemochromatosis** – a genetic disorder in which the body stores excess iron

323. **hemoglobin** - the oxygen-carrying pigment and predominant protein in red blood cells

324. **hemolysis** - destruction of red blood cells, resulting in the release of hemoglobin into the blood plasma

325. **hemophilia** – tendency to excessive bleeding, inherited by males through their mothers

326. **hemorrhage** – excessive flow of blood

327. **hemorrhoid** – swelling of the blood vessels in and around the rectum, resulting in burning, itching, painful discomfort

328. **hepatitis** – inflammation of the liver

329. **herniorrhaphy** – *(her-nee-or-a-fee)* surgical repair of a hernia

330. **heterochromia iridis** – condition where the iris of each eye is a different color, or one or both is flecked with a different color

331. **histiocytosis** - a rare but dreadful disorder with parallels to cancer, in which

332. one's own histiocytes (white blood cells also called macrophages) multiply and attack the very tissues and organs they were to protect

333. **homeopathy** – the practice of treating disease with drugs which, in a healthy person, would produce the same kind of symptoms as the illness

334. **humoral** – relating to the "humors" of the body, specifically the blood, lymph and inside the eyeball

335. **hyaline membrane disease** – a disorder of the lungs in newborns, especially premature infants, in which a glassy-looking membrane forms on the inside over the alveoli, making respiration difficult at best; now commonly known as respiratory distress syndrome (RDS)

336. **hydranencephaly** - a congenital condition in which the cerebrum of the brain is absent and replaced by sacs filled with cerebrospinal fluid; usually the cerebellum and brainstem are normal

337. **hydrocoele** – literally, "sack of water"; accumulation of fluid around the coating of the testis

338. **hygiene** – the activities associated with health, for instance, cleanliness

339. **hypercalcemia** – elevated levels of calcium in the blood

340. **hypercholesterolemia** – too much cholesterol in the blood

341. **hyperglycemia** – greater than normal level of sugar in the blood

342. **hyperplasia** – a condition resulting in an increase in the number of normal cells in an organ

343. **hypoglycemia** – lower than normal level of sugar in the blood

344. **hypoglossal nerve** – the 12th cranial nerve, which supplies the muscles of the tongue

345. **hypoplasia** – underdevelopment of an organ or tissue

346. **hypotension** – low blood pressure

347. **hypothalamus** – the area of the brain that controls body temperature, hunger and thirst

348. **hypothermia** – the lowering of body temperature below normal

349. **hypothyroidism** – underfunction of the thyroid

350. **hypovolemia** – abnormal decrease in blood plasma, resulting in lower overall volume

351. **hypoxia** – suffering from too little oxygen

352. **hysterectomy** – surgical removal of the uterus

353. **iatrapistic** – suspicious of physicians

354. **ichthyosis** - a group of skin disorders characterized by noninflammatory scaling of the skin and resembling fish scales

355. **idiopathic** – of unknown origin

356. **ileitis** – inflammation of the small intestine

357. **ileocolitis** – inflammation of both small and large intestines

358. **ileum** – the lower part of the small intestine

359. **ileus** – blockage of the small intestine, whether complete or not; causes constipation and bloating

360. **ilium** - the upper part of the pelvis, which forms the receptacle for the head of the femur at the hip joint

361. **immunodeficient** – lacking immune defenses

362. **immunoglobulin** – the protein actually involved in an immune response

363. **immunosuppression** – inhibition of the immune system

364. **in situ** – in the normal location

365. **in vitro** – literally, "in glass"; in laboratory settings

366. **in vivo** – in the body

367. **infarction** – death of an area of cells as a result of blockage from an embolus

368. **inguinal orchiectomy** – surgery to remove the testicle through an incision made in the groin

369. **intradermal** – within the skin layers

370. **intraperitoneal** – inside the peritoneum, or the body cavity

371. **intravenous** – inside the vein

372. **introitus** – an entrance into a canal or hollow organ

373. **intussusception** – prolapse (telescoping) of a portion of the intestine within itself, resulting in interruption of the blood supply, leading to an area of cell death and causing great pain; seen mainly in infants, boys more than girls, and unless diagnosed and corrected swiftly may be fatal

374. **ipsilateral** – on the same side

375. **ischemia** - inadequate circulation due to blockage of the blood vessels to an area

376. **ischium** – the lower part of the pelvic bone

377. **jaundice** – yellow tint of the skin and sclerae (whites of the eyes), caused by elevated bilirubin in the blood

378. **jejunum** – part of the small intestine, between the duodenum and the ileum (from the Greek word meaning, "empty", because upon death this part of the small intestine is always found to contain nothing

379. **jugular** – principle vein in the neck

380. **juxtaspinal** – next to the vertebral column

381. **karyocyte** – any cell having a nucleus

382. **keratectomy** – removal of part of the cornea

383. **keratoconjunctivitis** – inflammation in the eye, of both cornea and conjunctiva

384. **ketoacidosis** – in diabetes mellitus, the buildup of ketone bodies in the blood, accompanied by an

increase in acidity; a dangerous condition, it should be treated swiftly

385. **kyphoscoliosis** – "widow's hump", caused by deterioration of the spine

386. **labium** (pl. **labia**) - lip

387. **Lactobacillus acidophilus** – one of the "good" bacteria that normally help with digestion (if decimated by illness or antibiotics, can be easily replaced by eating yogurt containing "live cultures" of L. acidophilus)

388. **laparoscope** – device used to view the interior of the abdomen via a small incision in the belly

389. **laryngeal dystonia (dysphonia)** – voice disorder caused by involuntary spasms of the muscles in the larynx

390. **laryngectomy** – removal of part or all of the larynx

391. **larynx** – the "voice box"; located at the top of the throat, contains the vocal cords

392. **leiomyoma** – benign tumor of smooth muscle tissue

393. **leiomyosarcoma** – malignant tumor of smooth muscle tissue

394. **leukemia** – cancer of the blood

395. **leukoplakia** – white spot inside the mouth

396. **lingual** – of the tongue

397. **liposuction** – vacuum removal of body fat

398. **lobectomy** – removal of one or more lobes, as of the lung or thyroid

399. **longitudinal** – lengthwise, or durational

400. **lumbar** – relating to the lower back

401. **lymphangiogram** – x-ray of the lymphatic system

402. **lymphedema** – excess fluid in the lymph glands

403. **lymphocyte** – small white blood cell responsible for immune responses

404. **lymphoma** – tumor of the lymphoid tissue

405. **lysosome** – an organelle inside a cell that breaks down large molecules or bacteria taken in by the cell

406. **macerate** - to soften tissues after death by soaking and by enzymatic digestion, as happens with a stillborn child (do not confuse with *masticate*, to chew)

407. **macrobiotic diet** – one that claims to lengthen life, leaning chiefly on quantities of brown rice and vegetables; not recommended for pregnant women or children, and there is not enough protein included for some people's requirements

408. **macrophage** - type of white blood cell that ingests (takes in) foreign material; key players in the immune response to invaders such as infectious microorganisms

409. **macular degeneration** – loss of the ability to see straight ahead caused by breakdown of the macula

(central part of the retina) or invasion of it by blood vessels, especially common after age 60

410. **magnetic resonance imaging** – (MRI) a special radiology technique to view internal structures of the body using magnetism, radio waves, and a computer to produce the images of body structures

411. **malacia** – softening; for example, osteomalacia is the softening of bone (from a deficiency of calcium and vitamin D)

412. **malaria** - an infectious disease caused by protozoan parasites from the Plasmodium family that can be transmitted by the sting of the Anopheles mosquito or by a contaminated needle or transfusion (falciparum malaria is the most deadly type)

413. **malignant** - resistant to treatment or severe (e.g., malignant hypertension); in reference to a cancer, it implies the tendency to spread to other areas or organs of the body

414. **malleolus** – bony protuberances on either side of the ankle

415. **malleus** – one of the three bones of the middle ear ("the mallet"); the other two are incus and stapes *(stay-peez)*

416. **mammary gland** – the milk-producing gland within the female breast (the reason for breasts in the first place)

417. **mammogram** - an x-ray of the breast, taken with a device that compresses and flattens the breast, for the purpose of detecting abnormalities such as breast cancer; because of the discomfort and pain

associated with this procedure, women are sure it had to be invented by a man

418. **mandible** – the lower jaw

419. **mania** - an abnormally elevated mood state identified by the heightening of irritability, insomnia, speed or volume of speech, sexual desire, and energy or activity level, and by inappropriate elation, disconnected and racing thoughts, poor judgment, and inappropriate social behavior**manic-depression** - alternating moods of abnormal highs (mania) and lows (depression); called bipolar disease because of the swings between these diametrically opposed poles in mood

420. **marasmus** - wasting away from malnutrition, as in children who have kwashiorkor; also called **cachexia**

421. **masseter** – the muscle that raises the lower jaw

422. **mastectomy** – surgical removal of part or all of a breast, usually as a means of removing breast cancer

423. **mastitis** – inflammation of one or more of the mammary glands within the breast, usually experienced by a lactating woman

424. **mastoid** - the rounded protrusion of bone just behind the ear, once thought to resemble the breast (the name means "breastlike")

425. **maxilla** – the major bone of the upper jaw

426. **meconium** – dark, sticky material normally present in a baby's intestine at birth and passed in the feces

after birth; if passed before birth, this may be because of fetal distress

427. **medial** – nearer to the middle or center (opposite is lateral, to the side)

428. **median** – the middle itself

429. **mediastinum** - the area between the lungs, including the heart and its large arteries and veins, the esophagus, trachea, bronchi and lymph nodes

430. **Medicaid** – federally-funded state programs of public assistance to persons regardless of age whose lack the income and resources to pay for health care

431. **Medicare** - the US government's health insurance program for older people and some who are younger but disabled; funded by the Social Security Administration

432. **Medigap** - an insurance policy that supplements Medicare benefits and aims to fill the gaps in healthcare coverage

433. **medulla** – the innermost part (the term is not restricted to the brain)

434. **medulla oblongata** – the base of the brain, really a swelling at the top of the spinal cord, which controls breathing, blood flow and other essential functions

435. **megrim** – migraine; also refers to dizziness, vertigo or depression ("me grim" is very descriptive)

436. **melanin** – skin pigmentation produced by cells called melanocytes, which provides some protection again skin damage from the sun; melanin production

is increased in response to sun exposure (thus, tanning); freckles are small, concentrated areas of increased melanin production

437. **melanoma** – cancer of the melanocytes, usually visible at first as a spot that looks like a mole but has irregular borders or is an unusual color; melanoma can spread rapidly, but limited exposure to the sun and use of a high-SPF sunscreen can limit one's liability of contracting skin cancer in the first place

438. **melatonin** - hormone produced by the pineal gland, crucial to regulating the sleeping and waking cycles, among other processes

439. **membrane** – a thin layer of tissue that covers a surface

440. **menarche** – the onset of menstruation (puberty)

441. **meninges** (sing., **meninx**) – the three membranes that cover the brain (dura mater, pia mater and arachnoid)

442. **meningitis** – inflammation of the meninges, dangerous because it affects the brain

443. **meniscus** - a crescent-shaped structure, for example, the *medial meniscus* of the knee, a piece of cartilage which acts as a pad to ease movement of the joint

444. **menopause** – the cessation of menstruation, accompanied by hormonal changes; women experiencing menopause may be just as irritable as those undergoing menarche

445. **menorrhagia** – excessive bleeding at the usual time of menstruation which may also last longer than usual

446. **menstruation** – periodic shedding of the blood enriching the endometrium, the lining of the uterus which would have received a fertilized egg if one had happened along (also called *menses*, meaning literally "monthlies")

447. **mesentery** – tissue which attaches organs to the body wall, to keep them in place

448. **metabolism** – the entire range of chemical processes within the body, but used most often to refer to the digestion of food

449. **metacarpals** – the five long bones extending from the wrist to the fingers; the hand bones

450. **metastasize** – to spread, as a cancer

451. **methadone** – a synthetic opiate, used in some drug treatment programs as a legal substitute for heroin

452. **metrorrhagia** – uterine bleeding at irregular intervals

453. **microangiopathy** – thickening of the walls of capillaries to the point where they are weakened and bleed, leak protein, and slow the blood flow; diabetics may develop microangiopathy in many areas including the eye

454. **microcystic corneal dystrophy** - disorder in which the normally clear cornea shows dots (microcysts), tiny map-like lines, and grayish fingerprint lines on examination with a slit-lamp

455. **microtome** – a device used to cut extremely thin slices of tissue for examination under a microscope

456. **micturition** – urination, or the act of urinating

457. **migraine** – usually, periodic attacks of headaches on both sides of the head, often accompanied by nausea, extreme sensitivity to light, dizziness and impaired cognition

458. **milligram** – one thousandth of a gram; in the metric system, a gram equals the mass of one milliliter (one-thousandth of a liter) of water at 4°Celsius

459. **mimesis** – imitation, or mimicry; refers to the hysterical simulation of disease ("disease of the month"), or to one disease resembling quite another

460. **miosis** – contraction of the pupil (opp., *mydriasis*); do not confuse with **meiosis**, the process of chromosome replication

461. **mitchondria** – normal organelles located outside the nucleus within the cell, responsible for energy production

462. **mitosis** – normal division of a cell to form to new cells, each with the same genetic makeup as the original

463. **mitral valve** – (a.k.a. bicuspid valve)a valve with two flaps (cusps) situated between the left atrium and left ventricle of the heart; it permits blood to flow only from the left atrium into the left ventricle

464. **mittelschmerz** – *(mitt-el-shmerts)* pain between menstrual periods (from the German, literally "middle pain")

465. **MMR** – abbreviation for "measles, mumps, rubella", a universally administered childhood vaccine to protect against these three diseases

466. **molar** – grinding tooth, located toward the rear of the mouth

467. **Monilia** – yeast-like fungus now called Candida

468. **mononucleosis** – contagious infection with the Epstein-Barr virus (EBV, human herpesvirus 4), causing an increase of monocytes (white blood cells with a single nucleus); may be spread by saliva, thus the common term, "kissing disease"; manifested by fever, fatigue, sore throat and swollen lymph glands, mono can cause hepatitis and enlargement of the spleen

469. **monozygous twins** – twins from the same egg, always of the same sex and termed "identical"

470. **morbidity** – illness or disease

471. **morgue** – a place where deceased bodies are kept pending identification or autopsy

472. **morphine** – the main alkaloid in opium, used medically for pain relief; a powerful narcotic with strong analgesic action, it produces a false feeling of well-being and is dangerously addictive

473. **morphology** – form or structure, or the study of such

474. **mucosa** – referring to a mucous membrane, e.g., the oral mucosa (membrane inside the mouth)

475. **mucous** – the adjective that describes **mucus**, a thick fluid secreted by some parts of the body

476. **multipara** – the birth of more than one child at a time (twins, triplets, and so on)

477. **multiple myeloma** – malignant plasma cells (a form of lymphocyte), typically involving many sites in the bone marrow; also called *plasma cell myeloma*

478. **Munchhausen syndrome** – (moonch-how-zen) feigning of catastrophic illnesses, a psychological disorder marked by the insistence of the patient on treatment of an often dire illness that is, in reality, completely fictitious

479. **muscular dystrophy** – any of a group of genetic diseases involving progressive loss of the ability to control voluntary muscle movement; sometimes involuntary muscles, the heart and other organs may also be compromised

480. **mutism** – inability or unwillingness to speak

481. **myalgia** – muscle pain

482. **myelin** – the fatty covering of nerve cells

483. **myelogram** – an x-ray of the spinal cord and bones of the spine, made visible by a special dye

484. **myeloma** - tumor of plasma cells, antibody-producing cells that are normally found in the bone marrow

485. **myocardial infarction** – most commonly, a "heart attack", caused by the plugging up of any of the blood vessels of the heart; usually caused by

arteriosclerosis with narrowing of the coronary arteries, the triggering event being a clot (thrombosis)

486. **myocardium** – the heart muscle

487. **myoglobin** – the pigment in muscle that carries oxygen (related to *hemoglobin*, which operates in the blood)

488. **myometrium** – the muscular outer layer of the uterus

489. **myopia** – near-sightedness

490. **myxedema** – a dry, waxy swelling usually including swollen lips and nose; in infants, myxedema is also called *infantile hypothyroidism*

491. **narcolepsy** – a neurological disorder in which the sufferer suddenly has an overwhelming desire for sleep

492. **nares** – *(nair-eez)* the openings of the nostrils

493. **nasal septum** – connective tissue between the two passages of the nose

494. **nasogastric** – referring to the passage from the nose to the stomach

495. **nasopharynx** – *(nay-zo-fair-inks)* the area of the upper throat behind the nose

496. **naturopathy** - a system of therapy based on preventative care using mainly heat, light, water, air and massage; some practitioners use no medications at all, some recommend only herbal remedies, and a

very few who are licensed to prescribe may dispense pharmaceuticals when they feel the situation warrants

497. **nausea** – a feeling of queasiness, often a precursor to vomiting

498. **navel** – the umbilicus, or "belly button"

499. **nebulizer** – a device to administer medication in a fine mist into the nose; used particularly in ashthma patients

500. **necropsy** – autopsy; post-mortem examination

501. **necrosis** – cell or tissue death

502. **neonate** – newborn

503. **neophobia** – fear of anything new, innovation or change

504. **neoplasm** – literally, "new growth"; another word for a tumor

505. **nephritis** – inflammation of the kidney

506. **nephrosclerosis** – hardening of the kidney, usually because of the presence of arteriosclerosis (hardening of the arteries) which supply the kidney with blood

507. **neural** – referring to nerves

508. **neuralgia** – nerve pain

509. **neurodermatitis** - a general term for any itchy skin disorder thought to have emotional or "nervous" causes, e.g., an insect bite which, when scratched, becomes overly inflamed

510. **neuroma** – a tumor in nerve cells

511. **neurotoxin** – any substance that is poisonous to the nervous system; many insecticides are neurotoxins and should be handled with extreme care

512. **niacin** – nicotinic acid, one of the water-soluble B vitamins

513. **nictitate** – to wink

514. **nocturnal amblyopia** – "night blindness"

515. **nonpathogenic** – not causing disease

516. **nosocomial** - originating or taking place in a hospital, or acquired in a hospital, especially if an infection

517. **nucleus** - in cell biology, the structure that contains the chromosomes; in neuroanatomy, a group of nerve cells

518. **neutraceutical** – a food or part of a food that provides therapeutic or preventative benefits; *e.g.,* soybeans may be of benefit in preventing cancer and easing symptoms of menopause

519. **nystagmus** – rapid, repetitious, involuntary eye movements, may be horizontal, vertical or rotary

520. **obese** – grossly fat

521. **obstetrician** – a doctor concerned with the fetal development and delivery of an infant, and the accompanying care of the mother

522. **occiput** – *(ox-i-put)* the back of the head

523. **ocular** – of the eye, or of vision

524. **olfactory** – referring to the sense of smell

525. **oligospermia** – very little sperm (as in, a low sperm count – not real tiny ones)

526. **omentum** – a sheet of fat in the abdominal cavity covered by the peritoneum

527. **omphalocele** - a birth defect in which part of the intestine (sometimes the liver and spleen as well), covered by the amnion and the peritoneum, protrudes through an opening in the abdominal wall

528. **oncologist** – a physician who studies and treats cancer

529. **oophorectomy** – surgical removal of one or both ovaries

530. **ophthalmic** – pertaining to the eye

531. **orifice** – a natural opening in the body, e.g., ear, anus, nose, etc.

532. **oromandibular dystonia** – condition affecting the muscles of the jaw, lips, and tongue, in which the jaw may be pulled either open or shut, making speech and swallowing difficult

533. **orthopaedic** – literally, "straighten the child"; concerned with the repair and maintenance of the skeletal system (bones)

534. **orthoscopic** – correcting of vision

535. **oscitation** – yawning

536. **ossification** – deposit of calcium to form bone or bony tissue

537. osteomyelitis – bacterial infection of a bone, usually by deep injury or surgery

538. **osteopathy** – a form of treatment concerned with maintaining correct relationships between bones, muscles, and connective tissues; underlying thought is that as long as the body maintains proper relationship, it can heal itself; some practitioners do prescribe pharmaceuticals or chemotherapy

539. **otitis media** – inflammation of the middle ear

540. **otolaryngologist** – "ear, nose and throat" doctor

541. **oxygenation** – making oxygen available, either to tissues, the blood, or the patient himself

542. **oxytocin** – a hormone made in the brain that plays a role in both childbirth and lactation by causing muscles to contract in the uterus and the mammary glands in the breast

543. **paediatrics** – the medical treatment of children

544. **palliative care** – in one sense, palliative care means the steps taken to make the patient as comfortable as possible while not providing a cure, as in terminal

diseases; in another, this means providing only the barest minimum in a perfunctory manner

545. **palpebra** (pl., **palpebrae**) – the eyelid

546. **panacea** – cure-all; "magic bullet"

547. **pancreas** – an elongated, spongy organ located behind the stomach which aids in digestion and produces insulin to metabolize starches and sugars

548. **pandemic** – a widespread outbreak, usually of disease

549. **pantothenic acid** – vitamin B5, which is widely available in foods but still necessary for normal body function

550. **papilloma** – benign, clearly defined tumor that rises above the surface of the surrounding tissue; usually small and fairly round

551. **paralysis** – loss of function

552. **parasplenic** – located close to or alongside the spleen

553. **parenteral** - not enteric (via the intestine); *e.g.,* a substance administered by injection is parenteral

554. **parietal** – the side of the skull

555. **parotids** – salivary glands located in front of the ears

556. **paroxysm** – a violent attack

557. parturition – birth

558. **patella** – the kneecap

559. **pathogen** – agent causing disease

560. **pathology** – the study of disease; it is the pathologist who performs an autopsy

561. **pectoral** – referring to the chest

562. **pedodontics** – children's dentistry

563. **pellagra** – a condition caused by niacin deficiency, which if untreated proceeds from dermatitis, through diarrhea, to dementia and finally, death

564. **percutaneous** – through the skin

565. **perfusion** - a chemotherapy technique sometimes used when melanoma occurs on an arm or leg, in which a tourniquet is used to temporarily stop the flow of blood and anticancer drugs are put directly into the blood vessels of the affected area

566. **perinatal** – referring to the period encompassing just before birth and just after; can range from 20 to 28 weeks gestation to one to four weeks after birth

567. **periosteum** – a membrane of dense connective tissue that encases all bone except those parts in joints, which are covered by a synovial membrane

568. **peritoneum** – the membrane that covers the organs in the abdominal cavity

569. **pertussis** – whooping cough, a highly contagious, potentially deadly childhood disease

570. **petit mal** – refers to an epileptic seizure of moderate proportion (as opposed to *grand mal*, a severe seizure)

571. **phagocyte** – usually, a white blood cell that can engulf intruders in the bloodstream to protect the body

572. **phalanx** (pl., **phalanges**) – any of the bones in the fingers and toes

573. **pharingitis** – sore throat

574. **phenylketonuria** – (PKU) inherited inability to process the amino acid phenylalanine

575. **phlebitis** – inflammation of a vein

576. **physiatrist** - a physician specializing in physical medicine and rehabilitation, especially following trauma to the patient

577. **phytonutrient** – a beneficial compound found in plants, which may be important in preventing disease

578. **pineal gland** – a small organ located deep within the brain, believed to secrete melatonin, important in sleep regulation

579. **pituitary gland** – the main endocrine gland, located in the head, which secretes hormones that control virtually all the rest of the endocrine system

580. **placenta** – a temporary organ that supplies the developing fetus with nutrients from the mother and provides a repository for waste products from the

fetus; on birth, the placenta is expelled (the "afterbirth")

581. **plantar wart** – a flat wart that grows on the soles of the feet, caused by human papillomavirus; this wart invades the deep layers of the skin and can be very painful

582. **plasma** – the liquid part of the blood

583. **platelets** – irregular, disc-shaped structures in the blood that help in clotting

584. **pleura** – the thin covering that protects and cushions the lungs, made of two membranes with fluid between them

585. **pleurisy** – inflammation of the pleura; the pain from pleurisy can mimic the early signs of a heart attack

586. **pneumonia** – an infection that occurs when fluid and cells collect in the lungs

587. **pneumothorax** – free air in the chest, outside the lung

588. **podiatrist** – a doctor who treats foot abnormalities

589. **polio** – (abbr. for **poliomyelitis**) an acute and potentially devastating viral disease whose only natural host is man; the virus enters by mouth and multiplies in lymphoid tissues of the throat and intestine, then enters the blood and travels to other sites in the body where the virus community proliferates; eventually the central nervous system is compromised, with inflammation and accompanying loss of function (recovery may leave no effects, paralysis, or any degree between)

590. **polydactyly** – more fingers or toes than normal

591. **polyp** – a mass of tissue that develops on the inside wall of a cavity or hollow organ, such as the rectum

592. **porphyria** – any of a group of genetic conditions which include skin sensitivity to sunlight and/or by intermittent acute attacks of abdominal and nerve pain

593. **posteroanterior** – from back to front

594. **prepuce** – the foreskin of the penis

595. **presbyopia** – loss of the ability to focus on near objects, a result of aging

596. **proctology** – medical science concerned with the rectum and anus

597. **prophylactic** – general term for a preventive measure, not limited to condoms

598. **prostate** – a glandlike structure just beneath a man's bladder, which is actually composed of between 30 and 50 small glands, and which produces the seminal fluid that carries the sperm

599. **prosthesis** – an artificial substitute for part of the body (eye, hand, foot, tooth and so on), for functional or cosmetic reasons, or both

600. **proximal** – near

601. **psoriasis** – *(sore-eye-a-sis)* a hard, scaly rash on the knees, elbows, scalp, navel, genitals or buttocks, caused by the production of too much skin in those

places; thought to be an autoimmune disorder; some psoriasis victims also develop joint inflammation

602. **pulmonary** – relating to the lungs

603. **pustule** – a small boil or pus-filled sac

604. **quadriplegia** – the condition of being paralyzed in both arms and legs

605. **rectum** – the last several inches of the colon, where solid waste is stored until it leaves the body via the anus

606. **regurgitation** – backward flow, of food or blood

607. **renal** – of the kidney

608. **retina** – the rear part of the inside of the eye, on which images are focused

609. **rheumatology** – study and treatment of conditions of the musculoskeletal system and also the immune system

610. **rhinitis** – irritation of the nose

611. **rosacea** – redness and irritation of the skin on the face in areas where one would normally blush; tiny blood vessels in the skin enlarge and become inflamed; acne may appear, but rosacea is not treatable like normal everyday acne; the condition persists, and only with careful diet, limited exercise, avoidance of sun and antibiotics or cortisone can rosacea be controlled

612. **roseola** – a childhood viral disease seen mostly between 6 and 24 months of age, roseola is a red

rash that follows a very high fever, lasts 48 hours at most, then disappears; there are no apparent long-term effects

613. **rubella** – (German measles) a viral disease characterized by a rash of red spots beginning on the belly and spreading out; when a pregnant woman contracts rubella, her unborn child is at risk for a variety of birth defects and mental retardation

614. **saccharin** – an artificial sweetener which has been shown to be 300-500 times sweeter than sucrose

615. **sacrum** – the large, heavy triangular bone at the base of the spine, made up of fused sacral vertebrae

616. **sagittal** – lengthwise

617. **sarcoma** – a cancer that begins in bone or connective tissue

618. **scapula** – the shoulder blade

619. **sciatica** – pain resulting from irritation of the sciatic nerve, beginning in the lower back, traveling down the leg behind the knee and involving the entire lower leg

620. **sclera** – the tough, white outer covering of most of the eyeball

621. **scoliosis** – curvature of the spine

622. **sebum** – oil produced by the sebaceous gland, located around the base of a hair follicle, which preserves the flexibility of the hair

623. **sepsis** – "blood poisoning"; or, a blood stream infection

624. **serum** – the clear liquid that can be separated from clotted blood

625. **sesamoid bone** – a small bone embedded in a joint; the patella is a sesamoid bone

626. **sinus rhythm** – the normal regular rhythm of the heart, controlled by the sinus node

627. **somnambulist** – a "sleep-walker"

628. **sphygmomanometer** – *(sfig-mo-man-**om**-eh-tur)* a device used to measure blood pressure by means of an inflated cuff around the upper arm

629. **spina bifida** – a birth defect in which the spinal column fails to close properly

630. **spondylosis** – degeneration of the disc spaces between vertebrae

631. **squamous cells** – flat cells that resemble fish scales

632. **sternum** – the "breast bone"; the connection in the middle of the rib cage

633. **strabismus** – a condition in which the eyes appear to be looking in different directions; they may either diverge or converge (cross-eyes)

634. **sublingual** – under the tongue

635. **supine** – lying on one's back

636. **systole** – *(siss-toe-lee)* the time period when the heart contracts (as opposed to diastole, the resting period)

637. **tachycardia** – *(tacky-car-dee-ah)* rapid heart rate (more than 100 beats per minute)

638. **temporal** – of the temple, or the area of the head just above and in front of the ear

639. **thrombocyte** – a platelet

640. **thymus** – an organ behind the breastbone where lymphocytes mature and multiply

641. **tibia** – the larger of the two bones of the lower leg

642. **tinnitus** – "ringing in the ears"

643. **toxemia** – (pre-eclampsia, or preeclampsia) a condition that appears in the third trimester of pregnancy, involving a sharp rise in blood pressure (abrupt hypertension), leakage of large amounts of albumin into the urine (albuminuria) and swelling of the hands, feet and face (edema)

644. **trachea** – the "breathing tube" connecting the mouth and nose to the lungs

645. **tuberculosis** – a highly infections bacterial disease that involves mainly the upper respiratory system; TB is so virulent that the US Public Health Service mandates regular testing among the population (e.g., when a child enters school, when a person applies for a job, before surgery, and so on)

646. **tympanum** – the membrane commonly called the "ear drum"

647. **ureter** – a tube that connects the kidney to the bladder

648. **uvea** – part of the eye, including the iris, the choroid, and the ciliary body

649. **vena cava** – actually refers to two major veins: The superior (upper) vena cava is the large vein which returns blood to the heart from the head, neck and both upper limbs. The inferior (lower) vena cava returns blood to the heart from the lower part of the body.

650. **xanthoma** – yellowish, firm nodules in the skin which often point to hidden disease, such as diabetes, lipid disorder (hyperlipidemia) or other conditions; xanthoma is a harmless growth of tissue, but an indicator which should not be ignored.

You have reached the end of the audio review for
Medical Terminology.

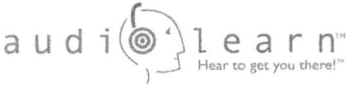

www.ingramcontent.com/pod-product-compliance
Lightning Source LLC
Chambersburg PA
CBHW070833180526
45168CB00002B/821